Ghassen Gader
Nesrine Jemel

Malignant Cerebral Meningiomas

Ghassen Gader
Nesrine Jemel

Malignant Cerebral Meningiomas

Diagnosis and therapeutic management

ScienciaScripts

Imprint

Any brand names and product names mentioned in this book are subject to trademark, brand or patent protection and are trademarks or registered trademarks of their respective holders. The use of brand names, product names, common names, trade names, product descriptions etc. even without a particular marking in this work is in no way to be construed to mean that such names may be regarded as unrestricted in respect of trademark and brand protection legislation and could thus be used by anyone.

Cover image: www.ingimage.com

This book is a translation from the original published under ISBN 978-620-6-71329-6.

Publisher:
Sciencia Scripts
is a trademark of
Dodo Books Indian Ocean Ltd. and OmniScriptum S.R.L publishing group

120 High Road, East Finchley, London, N2 9ED, United Kingdom
Str. Armeneasca 28/1, office 1, Chisinau MD-2012, Republic of Moldova, Europe
Printed at: see last page
ISBN: 978-620-8-17885-7

Table of contents

INTRODUCTION

Intracranial meningiomas are among the most frequent benign primary tumors of the central nervous system(1). The WHO defines three histological grades of meningioma according to their degree of malignancy (2). Grade III meningiomas are characterized by their rarity and aggressive behavior towards adjacent anatomical structures. They have a high risk of recurrence and a poor prognosis. The occurrence of neurological and extra-neural metastases has been described for this category of meningioma (3). There are 3 histological subtypes of grade III meningiomas: anaplastic meningioma, papillary meningioma and rhabdoid meningioma(4,5). These malignant meningiomas may be de novo or the result of degeneration of a low-grade meningioma.The clinical presentation of grade III meningiomas is nonspecific, and is characterized by a rapid progression of symptomatology.Despite the diagnostic contribution of brain MRI with multimodal sequences, distinguishing grade III meningiomas from other high-grade tumors can be particularly tricky in certain situations.

Treatment is based on surgery, with the aim of removing as much of the meningioma as possible in order to relieve compression on nerve elements and minimize the risk of recurrence. Adjuvant treatment (radiotherapy, chemotherapy) is discussed to improve the prognosis of these patients.

Early and appropriate treatment is necessary to guarantee a better quality of life and longer disease-free survival.

The objectives of our study were:

- Study the clinical and radiological presentation of grade III meningiomas.

- Evaluate the therapeutic management of these tumors.

- To study the prognostic factors and survival of patients managed for grade III meningioma with a comparison with data from the literature.

PATIENTS AND METHODS

1. POPULATION, TYPE AND PROCEDURE OF[i] STUDY :

II This is a retrospective, descriptive study of 15 patients operated on at the neurosurgery department of Ben Arous CTGB for grade III intracranial meningioma, over a period of8 years running from January 2014 to December2021.

1.1 Inclusion criteria:

The patients included were those operated on for intracranial meningiomas classified grade
III of (2), with anatomopathological confirmation on surgical specimen. All grade III meningioma subtypes (rhabdoid, papillary and anaplastic) were included.

1.2 Inclusion criteria :

Patients operated on for other extra-axial lesions were not included, in particular meningiomas of other grades, or lesions wrongly considered as meningiomas preoperatively and whose histological study suggested another lesion (meningeal metastasis, Rosai Dorfman disease).

1.3 Exclusion criteria :

Files were excluded in the event of missing data.

2. COLLECTEDESDONNEES :

We first drew up an information sheet, which identified the data to be studied from the patients' files. These data were then entered directly into a pre-established Excel spreadsheet.

2.1 Epidemiological and clinical data:

The following data were taken into account: age, sex, general condition according to the Karnofsky index (appendix 1) (6), medical and surgical history, association or not with neurofibromatosis type 2, reason for admission, duration of symptomatology before admission, and neurological examination on admission.

2.2 Radiological data :

They were collected from patients' preoperative brain CT and MRI scans. We studied:

Tumor location: skull base/ convexity/ para sagittal

Number and size

Radiological semiological characteristics

In patients presenting signs suggestive of secondary localization, an extension workup (CT-PET) was performed. The results of this work-up were noted.

2.3 Therapeutic data:

2.3.1 Surgery:
Medical preparation for surgery

Surgical approach

Technique of excision

Quality of excision: assessed with reference to SIMPSON classification (Appendix 2) (7)

Pathological data: macroscopic and microscopic study, immunohistochemical study. PART CHAPTER

Immediate and late postoperative complications.

2.3.2 Radiotherapy:
Total delivered dose

Dose splitting

Spreading the treatment

Total treatment time

2.3.3 Chemotherapy:
Type

Number of treatments.

Treatment duration

2.4 Evolutionary data :

Follow-up time

Notion of tumor recurrence

Notion of revision surgery

Survival times and cause of death.

3. ANALYTICAL STUDY :

The results obtained were presented in several forms:

Summary tables.

Histograms illustrating variations in the different variables.

Sector diagrams.

4. BIBLIOGRAPHICAL STUDY :

The bibliographic search was carried out on the PubMed, Science Direct,Google Scholar database using scientific articles published between 1996 and 2023, including systematic reviews, meta-analyses and case studies. The following keywords were used in the search: meningioma grade III, radiotherapy, neurosurgery.

5. ETHICAL CONSIDERATIONS AND CONFLICTS OF INTEREST :

Any information to be declared during or after the study will be in absolute anonymity. We declare that we have no conflict of interest in relation to this work.

RESULTS

1. EPIDEMIOLOGICAL STUDY :

1.1 Gender :

Our cohort comprised 15 patients: 5 (33%) women and 10 (67%) men, giving a sex ratio (M/F) of 2.

1.2 Age :

The average age of our patients at the time of diagnosis was 45 years, with extremes ranging from 3 to 78 years.

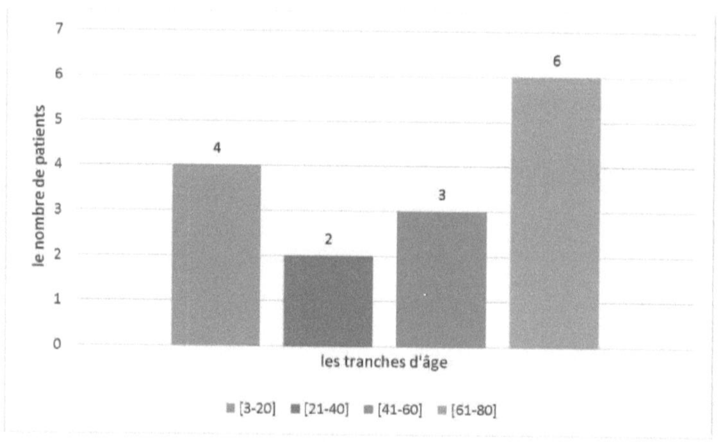

Figure 1: *Age distribution of patients*

The two most represented age groups are those under 20 and over 60.

1.3 History:

Inour series,8(53%) patients had a medical-surgical history:

Three patients were hypertensive

One patient was diabetic

One patient had breast cancer

Three patients had a history of cranial surgery for grade I or II meningioma:

A patient underwent surgery for a transitional meningioma (grade I) localized in the frontal parasagittal plane. He underwent SIMPSON III resection and received no adjuvant treatment postoperatively.

Two patients underwent surgery for atypical meningiomas (grade II). The 2 meningiomas were located in the convexity (frontal and parieto-occipital). Both patients underwent complete SIMPSON I resection, and received no adjuvant treatment.

- No cases of prior irradiation, use of synthetic progestins, or association with NF2 were noted in our study.

2. CLINICAL STUDY :

2.1 Diagnostic delay :

This is the time between the onset of clinical signs and hospitalization.

- Three patients were already known to have grade I or II meningiomas, and therefore subject to regular follow-up. The mean time from first cranial surgery to meningioma degeneration was 49.3 months.
- Five patients consulted us within a week of the onset of clinical signs.
- Three patients consulted within 1 week to 1 month.
- Four patients consulted us more than one month after the onset of clinical signs.

2.2 Reason for consultation :

- The main complaint that prompted consultation was a focal deficit found in 10 patients, representing 67% of cases in our series. This focal deficit is explained by the location of the meningioma and the consequent mass effect or infiltration of eloquent cerebral structures. These disorders were :

- o Motor symptoms such as heaviness in one hemicorpus in 7 patients.

  - o Visual disorders such as visual field amputation described in 2 patients

  - o Only one patient reported paresthesia of the lower limb.

- Signs of HTIC were present in 7 patients representing 47% of cases in our series. The main complaint was headache, more or less associated with nausea and vomiting.

- Epileptic seizures were noted in 4 patients (27% of cases in our series). In 3 cases, these were generalized tonic-clonic seizures, and in 1 case, partial clonic seizures of the upper limb. No patient presented with status epilepticus.

- Two patients (13%) consulted us because of the appearance of a curvature of the skull.

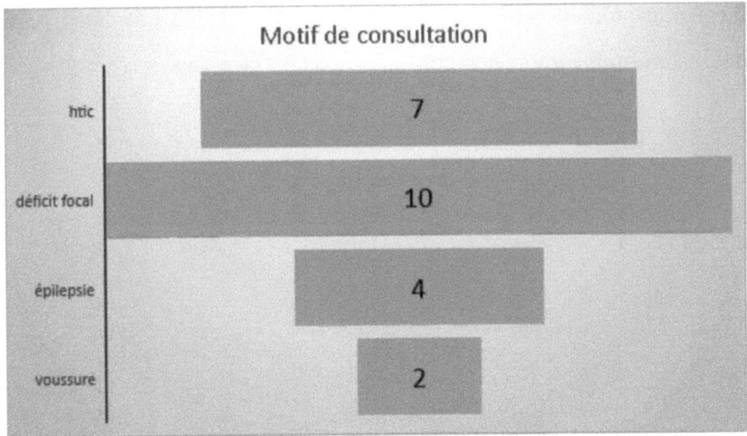

Figure 2: *Distribution of patients by reason for consultation*

2.3 **Physical examination :**

2.3.1 The Karnofsky index:

On examination, 5 patients were in good general condition, with a Karnofsky index of over 80%, while 10 patients were in average general condition, with a Karnofsky index of between 60 and 70%.

2.3.2 Neurological examination :

The neurological examination was normal in 5 patients. In the remaining 10 patients, the abnormalities detected during the examination were :

- HLH-type visual field amputation in 2 patients

- Hemiparesis in 5 patients, right in 3 cases and left in the other 2.

- Right kinetic cerebellar unsyndrome with nystagmus in 3patients

  - Involvement of the VIeme cranial pair, manifested by a right convergent strabismus in only one case.

2.3.3 Examination of the cephalic extremity :

In 2 cases, examination of the cephalic extremity revealed a rounded, hard, painless, non-mobilizable and non-inflammatory swelling.

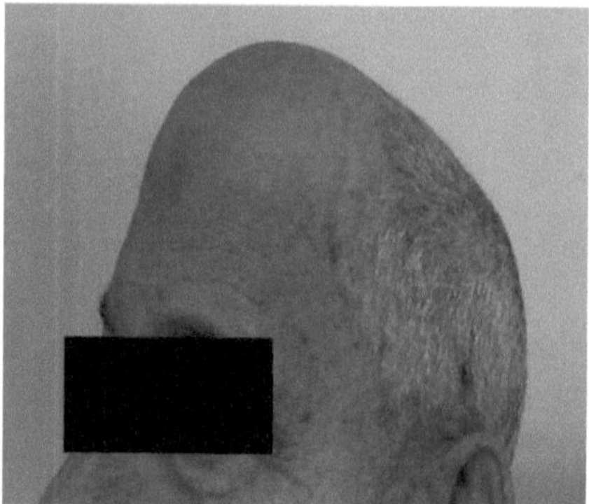

Figure 3:*Profile photograph of a patient with a left frontal arch*

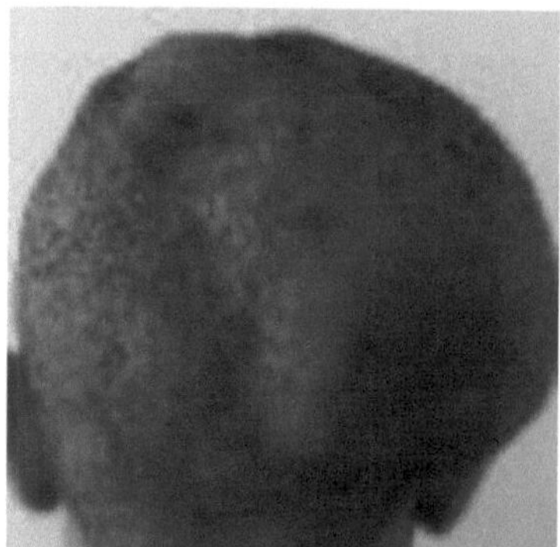

Figure 4: *Photograph of a patient showing a right parieto-occipital voussure*

3. **RADIOLOGICAL STUDY :**

3.1 **Cerebral CT** :

Performed preoperatively on 7 patients in our series.

3.1.1 *Density and contrast :*
The meningioma was isodense on non-injected brain CT in 2 patients, slightly hyperdense in 3 patients, and 2 other patients showed spontaneous hyperdensity related to stigmata of intra-tumoral bleeding. Contrast was homogeneous in 2 patients and heterogeneous in 5.

3.1.2 *Calcifications :*
Cerebral CT showed no spontaneous hyperdensities suggestive of calcifications.

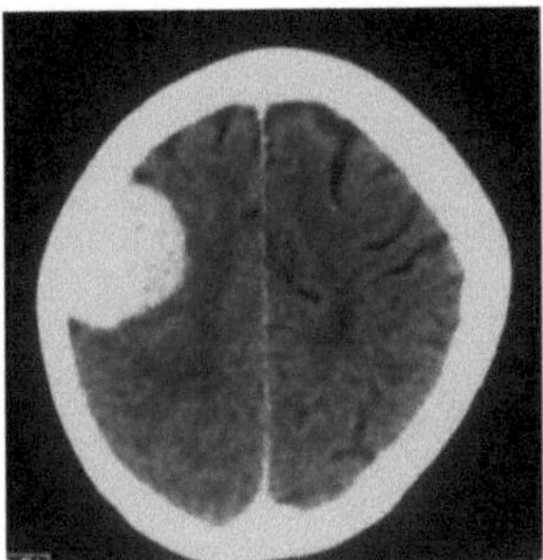

***Figure 5:**Axial section of a parenchymal CT scan with contrast injection showing a right frontal meningioma with intense, homogeneous contrast.*

3.1.3 *Bone involvement :*

Study of the bone structures in the corresponding windows revealed osteolysis in 3 cases, with extension of the lesion to the exocranial soft tissues.

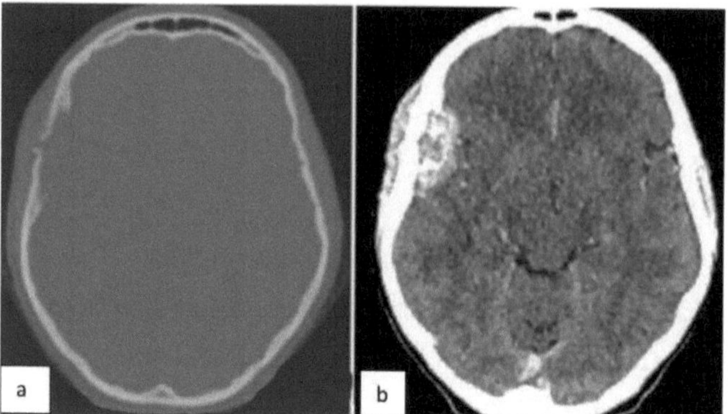

Figure 6:Axial sections of a CT brain scan in bone window (a) and parenchymal window with contrast injection (b) showing a right frontopteryngeal meningioma invading the adjacent bone.

3.2 Brain MRI:

All patients in our series underwent preoperative cerebral MRI, to better study the meningioma and its relationship with adjacent vascular and nervous structures.

3.2.1 Number of meningiomas :

Only one patient, who had previously undergone surgery for a right pterional meningioma, presented with meningiomatosis in connection with the coexistence of 4 meningiomas. However, he had none of the other Manchester criteria(8) for the diagnosis of NF2.

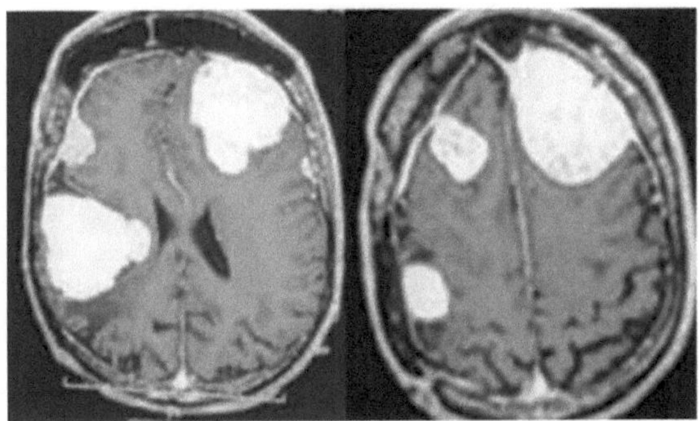

Figure 7: *Axial sections of a T1 sequence brain MRI with gadolinium injection showing meningiomatosis.*

3.2.2 Topography of meningiomas:

Grade III meningiomas were :

Parasagittal location in 6 cases, 3 of which invaded the lumen of the superior sagittal sinus

At convexity level in 6 other cases.

In 3 cases, the meningioma was located in the posterior cerebral fossa: 1 in the convexity and 2 in the cerebellopontine angle.

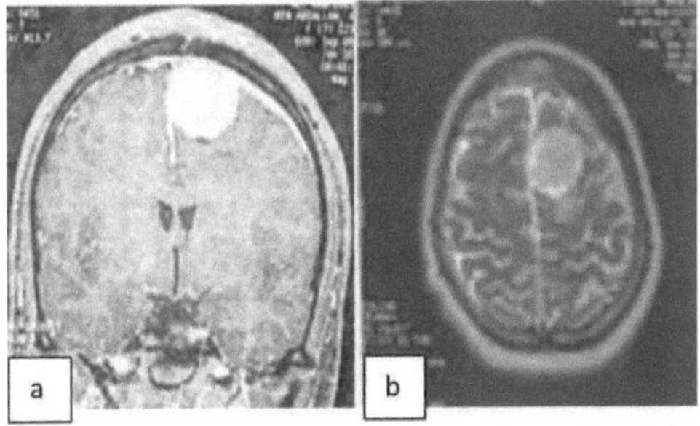

Figure 8:*Coronal (a) and axial (b) sections of a T1-weighted brain MRI with Gadolinium injection (a) and T2 (b) showing a parasagittal left meningioma.*

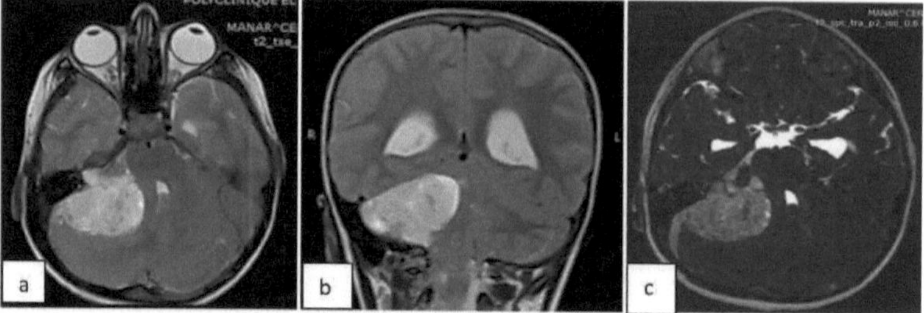

*Figure 9:**Axial (a, c) and coronal (b) sections of a T2-weighted (a, b) and Ciss-3D (c) brain MRI showing a right APC meningioma.*

3.2.3   Signal :

On T1 sequences, 8 patients had isosignal lesions, and a further 7 patients had hypersignal lesions.

T1 gadolinium contrast was homogeneous in 5 cases and heterogeneous in 10. The comet-tail sign was noted in 10 cases.

On T2 weightings, 6 lesions were isosignal, and 9 lesions were hypersignal.

Edema on the T2 FLAIR sequence was present in 13 out of 15 cases.

In 7 cases, the T2* sequence showed intra-tumoral bleeding.

Diffusion sequence and ADC showed diffusion restriction in 9patients.

Multimodal MRI with perfusion and spectroscopy sequences was performed in only 6 patients.

The perfusion sequence detected hyerperfusion in 4 cases and was inconclusive in the other 2. While the spectroscopy sequence showed in 5 cases a peak in choline, lipid and a fall in NAA and creatine.

The choline/creatine ratio was high. In 1 case, it was inconclusive.

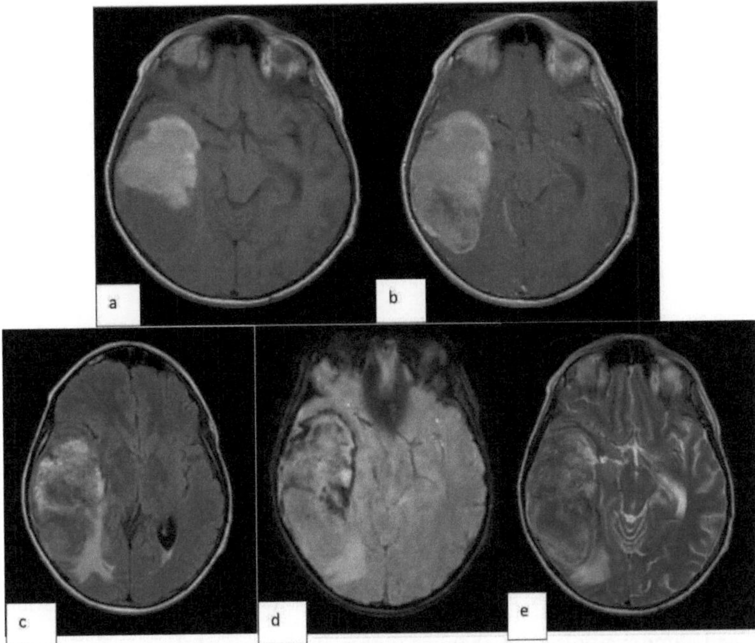

Figure 10:*Axial sections of a brain MRI in T1(a), T1 gadolinium (b), T2 Flair (c), T2*(d) and T2(e) sequence, showing a right temporo-occipital meningioma with stigmata of recent bleeding, associated with lesional edema and heterogeneous contrast.*

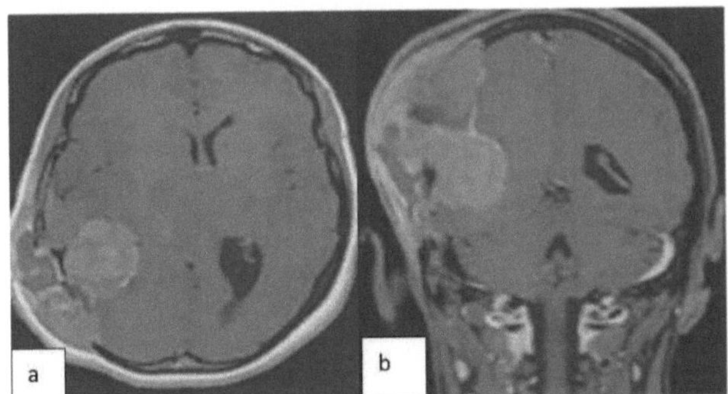

Figure 11:*Axial (a) and coronal (b) sections of a T1 brain MRI scan with degadolinium injection, showing heterogeneous contrast in a right parieto-occipital meningioma, with bone and skin invasion.*

3.2.4 Relationship with healthy parenchyma :

Brain MRI in all 13 patients showed infiltration of healthy brain parenchyma by the meningioma. The meningioma/parenchyma interface was blurred, with no CSF border visible on T2 sequences.

3.2.5 Meningioma size :

The mean size of the largest diameter of the meningioma on brain MRI was 47 mm, with extremes ranging from 80 mm to 25 mm.

3.2.6 Recurrence :

In our series, 3 low-grade meningiomas degenerated. This degeneration occurred in the same site as the previously operated lesion. Only one patient showed semio-radiological changes within the image of the recurrence of a grade I lesion, suggesting possible progression to a higher grade. These changes included significant peri-tumoral edema, "bumpy" tumor contours and heterogeneous contrast uptake.

3.3 Thoracoabdomino-pelvic CT :

TAP CT scans were performed in 3 patients with presenting signs of respiratory distress and altered general condition.

This examination detected pulmonary metastases in 2patients and a pharyngeal tumor in one patient.

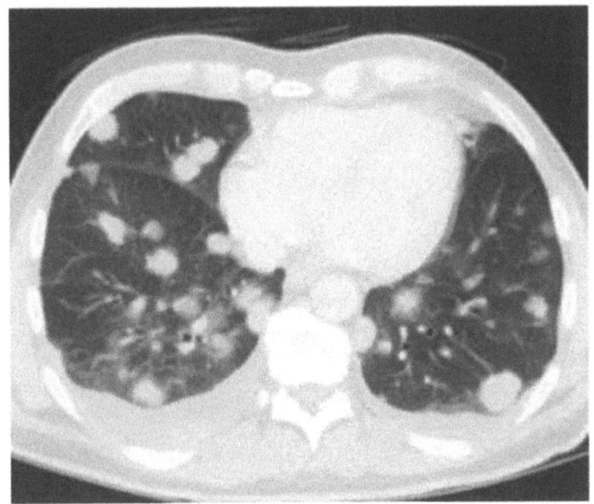

Figure 12:*Axial section of a thoracic CT scan showing multiple lung metastases*

4. THERAPEUTIC MANAGEMENT :

4.1 Preoperative management :

All patients received IV corticosteroids preoperatively to reduce peri-injury edema, relieve signs of HTIC, and optimize cerebral relaxation in preparation for surgery.

In addition to the 4 patients with preoperative epileptic seizures who were immediately started on antiepileptic drugs, all patients with a supratentorial meningioma were treated with anti-comitant drugs to prevent postoperative seizures.

4.2 Surgical management :
4.2.1   Time from admission to surgery:

The average time from admission to surgery was 5 days, with extremes ranging from 1 to 15 days. Only one patient underwent surgery 24 hours after admission, after presenting with an altered state of consciousness.

4.2.2   Surgical technique :

The aim of the surgery was to perform radical excision surgery. This was not possible in 11 cases:

- Hemorrhagic tumors in 3 cases.
- Proximity to vascular-nervous structures for the 6 para-sagittal meningiomas and the 2 APC meningiomas.

The surgical approach was adapted to the location of the meningioma:

Convex meningiomas, of which there were 6, were treated with a bone flap centred on the tumour.

In the case of a patient with meningiomatosis, only one lesion on the right parietal site was resected, given its large size, the mass effect it exerted and the associated peri-lesional oedema. The other lesions were inaccessible via the same approach.

For the 6 para-sagittal meningiomas. A flap exposing the superior sagittal sinus and the meningioma was used.

In the case of the cerebellopontine angle, a retrosigmoid approach was used in the 2 patients in question.

The posterior fossa convexity meningioma was operated on via a medial suboccipital approach.

Excision was performed by alternating removal of the meningioma and peripheral dissection of the healthy brain parenchyma.

The macroscopic appearance was that of a fleshy tumor, with a firm to elastic consistency found in all operated meningiomas. The color was whitish or grayish. Stigmata of intra-tumoral bleeding were present in 7 patients, and necrotic changes within the lesion were observed in 11 patients.

The dura mater and bone were sacrificed and replaced by dural plasty and cranioplasty in 2 cases.

Marked intraoperative bleeding was reported in 6 (40%) cases. These patients required intraoperative transfusion. This bleeding was controlled by coagulation, tamponade and suspension. This bleeding was of tumoral origin in 3 patients, and of venous origin in 3 patients with parasagittal meningiomas. The extent of this bleeding obliged the operator to perform partial exeresis in 3 cases of parasagittal meningiomas.

4.2.3   *Quality of surgical excision:*

The quality of surgical excision was assessed with reference to Simpson's grade:

- Twelve patients had a complete excision, with a Simpson score ranging from I to II.
- Three patients had exeresis deemed incomplete with a Simpson score of III and IV.

Parasagittal meningiomas were the main meningiomas for which excision was incomplete.

GràdeSimpson / Location	I	II	III	IV
Convexity	2	4	0	0
Parasagittal	0	3	2	1
Posterior fossa	0	3	0	0

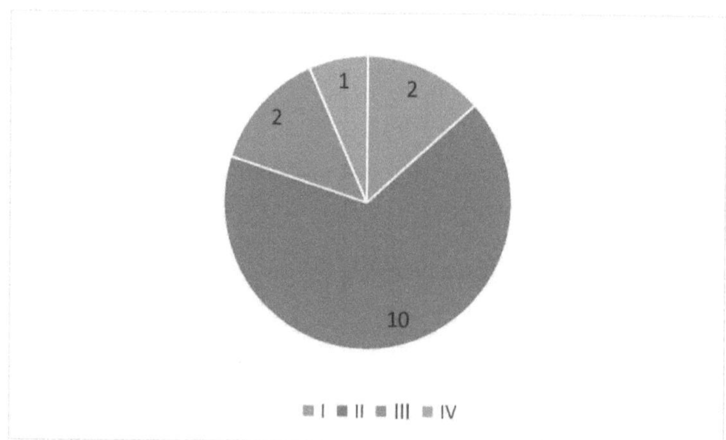

Figure 13: Distribution of patients according to the quality of excision assessed with reference to Simpson's classification

4.2.4   Post-operative complications

o <u>Early postoperative complications :</u>

During the first postoperative week, 4patients experienced postoperative complications:

Two of these patients experienced delayed awakening due to status epilepticus. Cerebral CT scans, routinely performed postoperatively in all patients, showed postoperative edemato-hemorrhagic remodeling, which did not necessitate repeat surgery. Seizures subsided after sedation and reinforcement of antiepileptic treatment. Patients were extubated an average of 48 hours after surgery.

One patient presented with pneumopathy, which was treated with antibiotics for 10 days with a favorable outcome.

A patient presented with swallowing disorders and facial paresis following excision of a cerebellopontine angle meningioma. He underwent gastrostomy feeding to control swallowing disorders. The patient kept the gastrostomy tube, given the lack of improvement in swallowing disorders. He died of septic complications related to his stoma 2 months after surgery.

o <u>Late post-operative complications (beyond one week) :</u>

Occurred in 2 patients:

One patient presented with a brain abscess 1 month after surgery. He was operated on again and received intravenous antibiotic therapy. After 2 weeks, he developed status epilepticus, requiring intubation, ventilation and

sedation. The patient showed no signs of waking up and died 10 days later.

A patient who presented with altered consciousness 2 weeks after surgery, in connection with bacterial meningitis and pneumopathy, with fatal outcome despite appropriate antibiotic therapy.

- One patient died 5 weeks after surgery.

Anatomopathological examination

In 12 cases, the meningioma was immediately classified as grade II:

Three cases of rhabdoid meningioma (20% of cases in our series)

Three cases of papillary meningioma (20% of cases in our series)

Six cases of anaplastic meningioma (40% of cases in our series).

Three other patients had already undergone surgery for a lower-grade meningioma. These cases are listed in Table 2 :

Table 2: Summary of previously operated and degenerated meningiomas

Patients	Initial histological type	Final histological type	Time from grade I/II to grade III	Location	SIMPSON of the first surgery
1	Atypical (grade II)	Rhabdoid	16 months	Parieto-occipital convexity	I
2	Transitional (grade I)	Anaplastic	96 months	Frontal parasagittal	III
3	Atypical (grade II)	Anaplastic	36 months	Frontal convexity	I

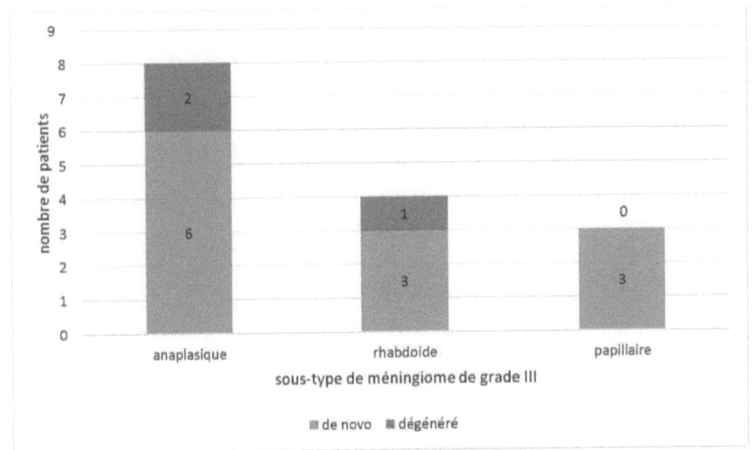

Figure 14: Distribution of patients according to histological subtype and de novo or degenerated nature

Immunohistochemistry was performed in 7 (47%) patients. EMA was positive in 4 patients. STTR2A and progesterone receptors were positive in 5. The mean Ki67 proliferation index was 30%, with extremes ranging from 20 to 48%.

No patient had a molecular biology study of their pathological specimen.

4.3 Radiotherapy :

Post-operative radiotherapy was indicated for all patients operated on after anatomopathological confirmation of the diagnosis of grade III meningioma. Only 8 patients underwent postoperative radiotherapy. The mean time to radiation was 6.5 months after surgery, with extremes ranging from 2 months to 14 months. Of the 7 patients who did not receive radiotherapy

Four died before the start of radiotherapy

A patient refused radiotherapy

Two patients had an altered general condition that was not compatible with radiotherapy.

No patient underwent stereotactic radiotherapy or radiosurgery. Doses ranged from 54 to 60 Gy, with an average of 56.5 Gy. Radiation therapy was conventionally fractionated and spread out (1.8 to 2 Gy per session, 5 sessions per week). Total treatment duration ranged from 5 to 7 weeks. The irradiation target volume included the tumor remnant if present, the operating bed and a margin of 1 to 2 cm, taking into account the persistence of malignant cells in the vicinity of the lesion site. Concerning late complications ? of radiotherapy, one patient reported asthenia with post-radiation alopecia. There were no cases of radionecrosis, neurocognitive disorders or hypopituitarism during the follow-up period.

4.4 Chemotherapy:

Three patients received adjuvant chemotherapy, indicated by the presence of extranedullary metastases. These patients had already undergone postoperative radiotherapy. The main molecules used were bevacizumab (targeted therapy!) and hydroxyurea. Bevacizumab was delivered to 2 patients at a dose of 5 mg/kg/14 days for 6 months. Only one patient received hydroxyurea at a dose of 20mg/kg for 3 months. Of these 3 patients, only one survived to the end of chemotherapy. No patient received hormone therapy.

5. EVOLUTION :

5.1 Overall survival :

The mean duration of postoperative follow-up was 22 months in our series, with extremes ranging from 1 to 51 months.

Only three patients survived beyond 2 years. All these patients underwent complete excision with radiotherapy.

Table 3: *Overall survival as a function of treatment*

Survival / Therapeutic protocol	<6 month	6 months and<1 year	1 year and <2 years	>=2 years
Complete excision with radiotherapy	0	1	3	3
Complete excision without radiotherapy	2	0	3	0
Incomplete excision with radiotherapy	0	1	0	0
Incomplete excision without radiotherapy	2	0	0	0

5.2 Tumor recurrence :

Seven patients experienced recurrence of their meningioma. Recurrence occurred after an average of 11 months in 5 patients awaiting adjuvant therapy. In the 2 other patients who underwent irradiation, tumor recurrence occurred after an average of 22 months following surgery. All these patients underwent re-operation, with a mean survival after re-operation of 20 months. Non-irradiated patients received radiotherapy after the second surgery.

Surgery on recurrent meningiomas was more delicate, given the areas adhered to by fibrosis and the great difficulty of individualizing the cleavage plane with the adjacent parenchyma. The quality of exeresis of the recurrence was judged SIMSPON II in 5 cases and SIMPSON III in 2 cases.

Table 4: Distribution of recurrences according to treatment

Simpson / Radiotherapy	I	II	III	IV
Yes (3)	0	1	1	0
No (4)	1	2	1	1

5.3   Metastases :

Four patients developed metastases postoperatively. Three of these patients had extra-neural metastases: 2 patients had secondary lesions in the lung ? and 1 patient had a pharyngeal metastasis. The mean time to onset of metastasis was 13 months after surgery. All patients underwent complete excision. Only one patient received radiotherapy for his meningioma postoperatively. Mean survival was 18.5 months. Table 5 summarizes the characteristics of these patients.

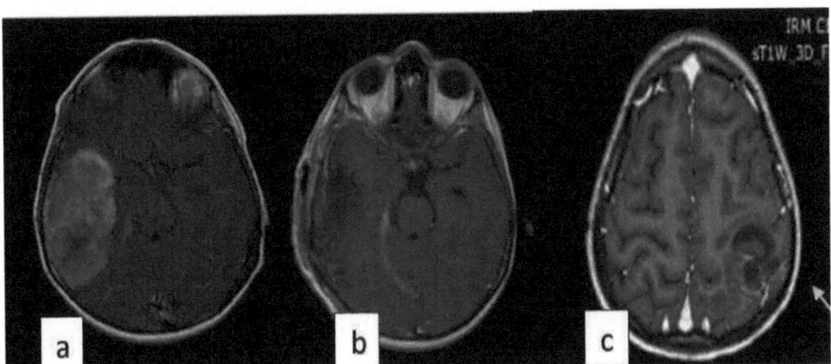

Figure 15: Axial sections of T1-weighted brain MRI with Gadolinium injection preoperatively (a), early postoperatively (b) and 3 months after surgery (c) showing complete removal of meningioma (b) and appearance of left rolandic metastasis (c)

Table 5: *Characteristics of patients who developed metastases*

Patients	Localization metastasis	Exeresis	Meningioma localization	Irradiation	Time to onset of metastases	Recurrence	Chemotherapy	Survival
1	Pharynx	Complete	Parasagittal	No	12 months	No	Yes	16 months
2	Lung	Complete	Parasagittal	No	10 months	No	Yes	17 months
3	Lung	Complete	Posterior fossa	No	10 months	No	Yes	15 months
4	Rolandique left	Complete	Convexity	Yes	20 months	No	No	26 months

DISCUSSION

1. EPIDEMIOLOGY :

1.1 Frequency :

Grade III meningiomas are rare. They account for 1.7% of all intracranial meningiomas(5,9). Their incidence is estimated at 0.12 per 100,000 population (10).

1.2 Age of discovery :

The incidence of meningiomas increases with age. Grade III meningiomas peak between 75 and 84 years of age, and decline from 85 onwards(5).

The mean age described in the series by Ruzevick et al. was 57.6 years (11); in our series, the mean age was 45 years.

1.3 Sex ratio :

The sex ratio for malignant meningiomas was 0.94(12) . While benign meningiomas have a much higher incidence in women, high-grade meningiomas occur almost twice as frequently in male subjects(13).In the literature, the sex ratio also depended on the age range of the patients.The incidence of grade III meningiomas was significantly higher in women in the 35-64 age group, while in the group of patients over 75, men were in the majority(5).

1.4 History and risk factors :

A history of cephalic irradiation increases the risk of developing meningiomas. Children who have been irradiated are 6 to 10 times more likely to develop a high-grade meningioma. The most affected are those who have been treated for scalp ringworm or acute lymphoblastic leukemia. These meningiomas can appear up to ten years after radiotherapy(14).

Progesterone acetate has also been implicated in the development of meningiomas, with no influence on histological grade. Discontinuation of treatment on discovery of the meningioma has led to cessation of growth and even regression of these lesions(15). In our series, there was no history of irradiation or use of progesterone acetate.

The association between meningioma and breast cancer has been widely described in the literature. The most frequently cited hypothesis is that a hormonal imbalance favors the appearance of the 2 pathologies. A recent discovery has shown that BRCA1 inactivation associated with the BAP1 suppressor gene is found in patients with rhabdoid meningioma. This loss of expression is correlated with a poor prognosis and a risk of rapid meningioma recurrence. This association between meningiomas and breast cancers is predictive of the development of rhabdoid meningiomas(14).In our series, we report the case of a patient presenting with an association between breast cancer and anaplastic meningioma.

It is estimated that 50-75% of patients with NF2 develop meningiomas, which are often grade II or III. The prognosis is poorer, with a higher rate of recurrence (16).None of the patients in our series were NF2 carriers.

2. CLINICAL STUDY :

2.1 Diagnostic delay

In equal proportions, grade III meningiomas may develop de novo, or result from anaplastic degeneration of another, lower-grade meningioma (4).

2% of grade I meningiomas and 15% of grade II meningiomas progress to grade III meningiomas. The average time between surgery and degeneration into malignant meningioma is 5.7 years for grade I and 1.4 years for grade II(17).

2.2 Clinical symptoms

There are no specific signs for grade III meningiomas. Rather, it is the rapid evolution of the clinical picture that is suggestive of malignancy. Neurological signs vary according to the location of the meningioma, with epilepsy a frequent consequence of peri-lesional edema and infiltration of healthy parenchyma (18). Rapidly progressive cranial voussures may, although not specific, point to this diagnosis(19).

3. RADIOLOGICAL STUDY :

3.1 Brain CT

Compared to "classic" meningiomas, malignant forms show alarming CT features: presence of haemorrhage, heterogeneous contrast, excessive oedema, osseous changes in the direction of osteolysis with a tendency to exocranial extension(20)   .   Certain   localizations,   in Toccurrenceparasagittaland fronto-parietal, are more frequently associated with a higher histological grade(21).

3.2 Brain MRI

Cerebral MRI plays an important role in the study of meningioma characteristics and their relationship with adjacent vascular and neural structures, especially for malignant variants that are deliberately more aggressive towards adjacent vascular and neural structures.

Certain semiological features are predictive of high-grade meningioma. These include necrosis or intratumoral haemorrhage. Cerebral edema, which can be seen in benign meningiomas, is deliberately more extensive in malignant forms, and the T1-hyposignal CSF line, reflecting the arachnoid plane at the meningioma/parenchyma interface, is classically absent. Frequent invasions of bone and skin are also noted, as are irregular tumor contours(22).

The advent of multimodal MRI has made it easier to distinguish between benign and high-grade meningiomas(23). ADC restriction on the diffusion sequence is a good indicator of meningioma malignancy (24). The perfusion sequence also shows hyperperfusion in malignant meningiomas. A comparison of the rCBV of the meningioma and the peritumoral edema can be of great help (25). The value of spectroscopy in the diagnosis of high-grade meningiomas is debatable. Some authors consider that this method does not clearly distinguish between high-grade and low-grade meningiomas, while others indicate that the presence of lactate or lipid peaks could be an indicator of meningioma malignancy (26,27).

Differential diagnosis

Problems of preoperative diagnosis are common for extra-axial lesions showing signs of malignancy. These include, but are not limited to, solitary fibrous tumors, glioscarcomas, leiomyosarcomas and meningeal metastases(19). Despite the decisive contribution of multimodality radiological techniques, a definitive diagnosis can only be made on the basis of histological and immunohistochemical studies on excisional specimens or tumour biopsies.

4. PRISEEN CHARGETHERAPEUTIC :

4.1 Surgical treatment

Surgery is the main treatment for meningiomas. Common principles of surgical technique apply irrespective of the grade and location of the meningioma:

- Craniotomy centered on the meningioma, exposing as much of the dural insertion base as possible, optimized by neuronavigation

- Early devascularization of the tumor by approaching the insertion base

- Excision alternating between a central cut and progressive peripheral dissection of the cleavage plane with healthy parenchyma, while controlling haemostasis. Removal of pathological dura mater and invaded bone is desirable whenever possible.

Surgery is the reference treatment for grade III meningiomas, with the aim of achieving the most complete exeresis possible. The SIMPSON(7) classification remains the reference method for describing the extent of excision. It is determined by the surgeon and by postoperative imaging. The extent of excision is the most important predictor of local control and progression-free survival, independently of tumour grade and other prognostic factors (14).however, some authors have shown that the quality of surgical excision of grade III meningiomas improves survival only moderately. There was no statistically significant difference in survival between patients who underwent Simpson I and inferior exeresis(28).

Post-operative complications of malignant meningiomas are numerous, given the frequent invasion of parenchyma, bone and skin, making exeresis laborious, delicate and prolonging operative time. In the literature, in a series of 63 patients, 10% presented medical complications and 31% complications directly linked to surgery: prolonged coma, dysphagia, neurological deficits(29).

4.2 Anatomopathological study :

The WHO classification of grade III meningiomas has undergone some modification, especially in 2021 with the advent of molecular biology (30). Diagnostic criteria since the WHO classification of 2000 include a mitosis count of 20 or more per 10 fields (x400) on light microscopy, or frank histological signs of anaplasia with pseudo-sarcomatous, pseudo-carcinomatous or pseudo-melanomatous histology(2). 50% of grade III meningiomas are anaplastic. The other 2 subtypes, papillary and rhabdoid, are considered when there is a successive majority papillary or rhabdoid component:

Rhabdoid meningiomas feature eccentric nuclei with a large nucleolus and cytoplasm containing an eosinophilic para-nuclear inclusion.

Papillary meningiomas are characterized by perivascular pseudopapillae: loss of cohesion with perivascular gathering of tumor cells, and perivascular spaces devoid of nuclei (2).

Immunohistochemistry is not routinely used for diagnostic purposes, especially as there is currently no specific marker for grade III meningiomas.

Loss of progesterone receptor expression is common in grade III meningiomas, which may also express "abnormal" markers such as cytokeratins(31). The Ki-67 proliferation index correlates well with meningioma grade. However, it has not been validated by the WHO, due to reproducibility difficulties. It remains the most widely studied and routinely used prognostic marker. In the literature, the Ki-67 index is an independent prognostic factor associated with progression-free survival and overall survival. Patients with lower-grade meningiomas whose index is greater than 20% have a survival similar to that of patients with grade III meningiomas (32).

4.3 Radiotherapy

Radiotherapy is the adjuvant treatment of choice following surgery to remove a grade III meningioma, whatever the quality of removal(33). According to Dziuk, progression-free survival at 5 years is 80% for grade III meningiomas treated by complete removal (Simpson I and II) with adjuvant radiotherapy. With resection of similar quality but without radiotherapy, progression-free survival drops to 50%(34).

Several techniques are used to irradiate high-grade meningiomas(35) :

- Conformal radiotherapy (with or without intensity modulation)
- Stereotactic irradiation, such as radiosurgery and stereotactic hypofractionated radiotherapy.

The technique that has proved most effective is conformal radiotherapy, with a preference for intensity modulation to limit radiation toxicity (35). The authors recommend a total dose of 60 Gy in fractions of 1.8 to 2 Gy per session, 5 days out of 7, over 5 to 7 weeks (35). Radiotherapy should be administered as soon as the surgical scar has consolidated(34). Some authors have studied the benefit of increasing the dose administered beyond 60Gy, given the aggressive nature of meningiomas(36) . Results remain inconclusive (30).

The target volume includes the tumour remnant if present, the operating bed and a margin of 1 to 2 cm to allow for microscopic meningeal disease. Margins are larger for meningeal extensions and any bone invasion, and smaller for the brain(35).

Stereotactic hypofractionated radiotherapy is mainly indicated for lesions close to the optic tract, with irradiation doses ranging from 20 Gy to 30 Gy at 80% isodose in 3 fractions, and from 25 Gy to 40 Gy at 80% isodose in 5 or more fractions. The target tumor volume varies from one team to another, with discrepancies concerning whether or not to include the comet tail in the· irradiation volume(35).

Radiosurgery has not demonstrated a clear benefit in the overall survival and remissions of malignant meningiomas (4).

The most frequent complications encountered after conformal radiotherapy are radiation-induced edema, asthenia, vertigo, skin erythema and cognitive impairment. For hypofractionated stereotactic radiotherapy, complications are very rare. No prophylactic drug treatment is recommended following irradiation(35).

4.4 Systemic treatment :

Chemotherapy and immunotherapy are indicated as palliative treatments. However, their efficacy remains open to debate (37). Their main field of application concerns recurrences with no local treatment option, and distant metastases.

Cytotoxic agents have not proved effective. On the other hand, following the study of genetic alterations in meningiomas, targeted therapy, in particular with anti-angiogenic agents, has shown promising results in the palliative treatment of malignant forms (33). Somatostatin analogues and hormone therapy have shown limited efficacy. In contrast, tyrosine kinase inhibitors and monoclonal antibodies, particularly those targeting angiogenic signaling such as sunitinib and bevacizumab, have shown promising results.

Immune checkpoint inhibitors such as ipilimumab, nivolumab, pembrolizumab and avelumab have also shown encouraging results in some patients (38).

4.5   Decision tree :

Given the rarity of grade III meningiomas, there are currently no publications with a high level of evidence or large randomized studies to prioritize the management of these lesions. A decision tree was proposed in 2020 by the French National Cancer Institute, as a rough guide to more robust treatment protocols and regimens(35).

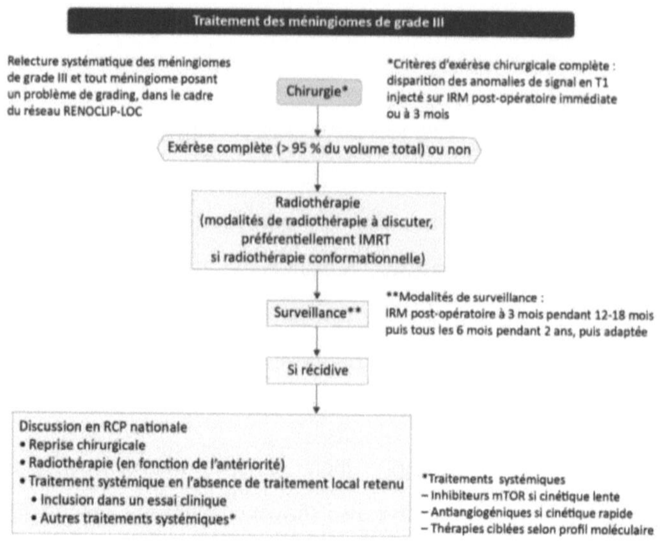

Figure 16: *Decision tree for the management of grade III malignant meningiomas proposed by the French National Cancer Institute (35)*

5. EVOLUTION AND PROGNOSTIC FACTORS :

5.1 Recurrences :

Malignant meningiomas have a higher and earlier recurrence rate than low-grade meningiomas. Despite advances in surgical and radiotherapy treatment, recurrence rates vary between 50% and 94% at 5 years (39).

Monitoring is performed by MRI of the brain immediately after surgery, at 3 months for 1 year and then every 6 months thereafter. This regimen can be customized on a case-by-case basis, depending on the clinical situation, tumor remnant and disease progression kinetics(35). The reference treatment in this case is surgical revision. Sughrue has shown that the mean survival after revision surgery for recurrent Grade III meningioma is 53 months, whereas without surgery, the mean survival is 25 months (25).

5.2 Metastases :

The appearance of metastases marks a pejorative evolutionary turning point in the history of malignant meningiomas (40). Their frequency is estimated at 8.9% (41,42).the mechanism of formation of neuraxial metastases is thought to be related to dissemination via the CSF. While a hematogenous origin through invasion of the venous system seems to be the cause of systemic metastasis. This explains why metastases are frequent in parasagittal meningiomas (34). Although there is no consensus on the systematic performance of a TAP CT scan for grade III meningiomas, some authors suggest that patients undergoing surgery for grade III meningiomas should be systematically screened for metastases as early as the first surgery. Their rationale is that early diagnosis of a single metastasis in an asymptomatic patient has a better prognosis than in patients with multiple metastases (33). Screening is carried out by TAP CT or FDG PET scan, or ideally by DOTATOC(43). Although the lungs are the most frequent site of metastasis, other localizations such as liver, bone and subcutaneous tissue have been described (4). Risk factors for metastasis include a history of previous meningioma surgery, invasion of the venous system by the meningioma and multiple recurrences (44).

5.3   Survival and prognosis:

Patients with grade III meningiomas, even after radiotherapy and systemic treatment, have a mean progression-free survival of 3.6 months ?and an overall survival of 23 months (45).

In contrast to the evolutionary pattern described for glioblastomas, with a more favorable evolution for mutant than wild-type genotypes, de novo anaplastic meningiomas have better survival rates and later recurrence times than degenerate meningiomas (11). In a series of 52 patients, Peyre demonstrated that overall survival for de novo grade III meningiomas was 3.1 years, while it was 2.1 years for degenerate meningiomas.

Good prognostic factors according to the literature are :

- Complete exeresis
- Young age
- Reduced tumor volume
- The Caucasian race
- Adjuvant radiotherapy
- Low levels of KI-67/MIB-1.

The location of the meningioma is also a prognostic parameter. Indeed, meningiomas located in the convexity and lateral part of the skull base often have a Ki-67 rate of over 4%, higher than those located in the medial part of the skull base (46).

CONCLUSIONS

Grade III meningioma is a rare tumor accounting for 1.7% of all meningiomas (5). Three histological subtypes exist: anaplastic meningioma, papillary meningioma and rhabdoid meningioma. The incidence of these meningiomas is higher in women in the 35-64 age group, while in the group of patients over 75, men predominate (5). Malignant meningiomas may be single or multiple in the context of NF2 (16). Grade III meningiomas may present with HTIC, epilepsy, focal deficit or cranial curvature. Radiological diagnosis is based on cerebral CT scan, but above all on cerebral MRI, which allows us to suspect a high-grade meningioma. A thoraco-abdomino-pelvic CT scan is sometimes necessary to assess the extent of the disease. Surgical excision, as complete as possible, followed by adjuvant radiotherapy, is the standard treatment. In some cases, surgery is a challenge, given the meningioma's vascular-nerve relationships.

We performed a retrospective study involving 15 patients operated on at the neurosurgery department of the CTGB in Ben Arous for grade III intracranial meningioma, over a period of8 years (January 2014 to December2021).

Our aim was to study the different clinical, radiological and therapeutic presentations of TOMS grade III meningiomas, and to evaluate survival time according to the proposed therapeutic protocols in comparison with the literature.

The mean age of our patients was 45 years. There were 5 women and 10 men, with a sex ratio of 2. Three patients had a history of cranial surgery for grade I or II meningioma. Only one patient had meningiomatosis without a history of NF2. Only one patient had a history of breast cancer. No previous irradiation or use of synthetic progestins was noted in our study. The main complaint of our patients was a focal deficit present in 10 patients. Signs of HTIC were present in 7 patients, epileptic seizures in 4 patients and 2 patients had cranial voussure. The examination revealed a Karnofsky index greater than 80% in 5 patients, while the other 10 patients had a Karnosfky index between 60 and 70%. The neurological examination was pathological in 10 patients. HLH was present in 2 patients, hemiparesis in 5 patients, kinetic cerebellar syndrome with nystagmus in 3 patients, and involvement of the 6th cranial pair in only 1 patient. Two patients had a rounded, hard, painless, non-mobilizable cranial swelling. Cerebral CT scans were performed in 7 patients, while MRI scans were performed in all.

The meningioma was located parasagittally in 6 cases, and convexly in 6 others. In 2 cases, the meningioma was located in the APC and in 1 case in the convexity of the posterior fossa. Cerebral MRI contrast was heterogeneous in 10 cases, with perilesional edema present in 13 out of 15. Multimodal MRI was performed in 6 patients. It showed hyperperfusion in the perfusion sequence in 4 cases. Spectroscopy showed choline and lipid peaks and a fall in NAA and creatine in 5 cases. The choline/creatine ratio was high. In 1 case, it was inconclusive. Three patients underwent TAP CT scans for signs of extranedullary metastases.

All our patients underwent excision surgery, with complete excision in 12 cases deemed SIMPSON I or II. Pathological examination revealed 4 rhabdoid meningiomas, 3 papillary meningiomas and 8 anaplastic meningiomas.

Eight patients underwent postoperative external conformal radiotherapy with intensity modulation on the tumor bed. A mean dose of 56.5 Gy was delivered in fractions of 1.8 and 2 Gy per session over 5 to 7 weeks. One patient reported asthenia with post-radiation alopecia. Patients who did not undergo radiotherapy either opted out of adjuvant treatment, had an altered state of health or died before radiotherapy.

The average follow-up time after surgery was 22 months. Seven patients experienced recurrence of their meningioma. Recurrence occurred after an average of 11 months in 5 patients awaiting adjuvant treatment. In the other 2 patients who underwent irradiation, tumour recurrence occurred after an average of 22 months following surgery, and all these patients underwent re-operation, with an average survival after re-operation of 20 months. Four patients developed metastases after an average of 13 months post-surgery. Three patients had extranedullary metastases and one had a brain metastasis. All three patients received chemotherapy. The main molecules were bevacizumab and hydroxyurea. Only one patient survived after chemotherapy.

During the follow-up period, only three patients survived beyond 2 years. All these patients underwent complete excision with radiotherapy.

Discussion of these data from the literature has led to the conclusion that the prognosis for grade III meningiomas is unfavorable. The risk of recurrence is high, and metastases are possible. Several prognostic factors have been identified to predict the outcome of these patients. These include young age, female gender, good initial general condition, complete resection and low KI 67%(35).

Despite the development of diagnostic and therapeutic methods, the prognosis of grade III meningiomas remains poor. A nationwide effort is needed to improve the time to treatment, which will improve survival.

APPENDICES

Appendix 1: Karnofsky(6) classification of general condition

Index	Description
100	Normal; no complaints, no signs of illness.
90	Able to pursue normal activity; minor signs or symptoms of illness.
80	Normal activity, with effort; some signs or symptoms of illness.
70	Autonomous; unable to carry on a normal activity or work actively.
60	Occasional need for assistance but able to provide for basic needs.
50	Considerable need for personal assistance, frequent medical care.
40	Invalid; need for specific care and assistance.
30	Completely disabled; indication for hospitalization, no imminent risk of death.
20	Very ill; hospitalization required, active or supportive treatment

	necessary.
10	Moribund; fatal outcome near.
0	Deceased.

Appendix 2: SIMPSON classification(7)

Surgical exeresis quality according to SIMPSON	
Grade1	Complete resection of lesion, including dura mater and normal bone
Grade2	Complete resection with labasedural coagulation
Grade3	Coagulation-free resection of the dural base
Grade4	Total resection
Grade5	Simple decompression, biopsy

BIBLIOGRAPHY

1. Ostrom QT, Cioffi G, Gittleman H, Patil N, Waite K, Kruchko C, et al. CBTRUS Statistical Report: Primary Brain and Other Central Nervous System Tumors Diagnosed in the United States in 2012-2016. Neuro-Oncol. Nov 1, 2019;21(Supplement_5):v1-100.

2. Louis DN, Perry A, Reifenberger G, von Deimling A, Figarella-Branger D, Cavenee WK, et al. The 2016 World Health Organization Classification of Tumors of the Central Nervous System: a summary. Acta Neuropathol (Berl). June 2016;131(6):803-20.

3. Wen PY, Packer RJ. The 2021 WHO Classification of Tumors of the Central Nervous System: clinical implications. Neuro-Oncol. August 2, 2021;23(8):1215-7.

4. Fountain DM, Young AMH, Santarius T. Malignant meningiomas. Handb Clin Neurol. 2020;170:245-50.

5. Kshettry VR, Ostrom QT, Kruchko C, Al-Mefty O, Barnett GH, Barnholtz-Sloan JS. Descriptive epidemiology of World Health Organization grades II and III intracranial meningiomas in the United States. Neuro-Oncol. August 2015;17(8):1166-73.

6. Mor V, Laliberte L, Morris JN, Wiemann M. The Karnofsky Performance Status Scale. An examination of its reliability and validity in a research setting. Cancer. May 1, 1984;53(9):2002-7.

7. Simpson D. THE RECURRENCE OF INTRACRANIAL MENINGIOMAS AFTER SURGICAL TREATMENT. J Neurol Neurosurg Psychiatry. Feb 1957;20(1):22-39.

8. Evans DGR, Baser ME, O'Reilly B, Rowe J, Gleeson M, Saeed S, et al. Management of the patient and family with neurofibromatosis 2: a consensus conference statement. Br J Neurosurg. Feb 2005;19(1):5-12.

9. Ogasawara C, Philbrick BD, Adamson DC. Meningioma: A Review of Epidemiology, Pathology, Diagnosis, Treatment, and Future Directions. Biomedicines. March 21, 2021;9(3):319.

10. Dolecek TA, Dressler EVM, Thakkar JP, Liu M, Al-Qaisi A, Villano JL. Epidemiology of meningiomas post-Public Law 107-206: The Benign Brain Tumor Cancer Registries Amendment Act. Cancer. 2015;121(14):2400-10.

11. Ruzevick J, Gibson A, Tatman P, Emerson S, Ferreira M. WHO grade III meningioma: De novo tumors show improved progression free survival as compared to secondary progressive tumors. J Clin Neurosci. Sept 2021;91:105-9.

12. Epidemiology for primary brain tumors: a nationwide population-based study | Journal of Neuro-Oncology [Internet]. [cited 28 Jan 2024]. Disponible sur: https://link.springer.com/article/10.1007/s11060-016-2318-3

13. Jaaskelainen J, Haltia M, Laasonen E, Wahlstrom T, Valtonen S. The growth rate of intracranial meningiomas and its relation to histology. An analysis of 43 patients. Surg Neurol. August 1, 1985;24(2):165-72.

14.   Wilson TA, Huang L, Ramanathan D, Lopez-Gonzalez M, Pillai P, De Los Reyes K, et al. Review of Atypical and Anaplastic Meningiomas: Classification, Molecular Biology, and Management. Front Oncol. 20 Nov 2020;10:565582.

15.   Champeaux-Depond C, Weller J, Froelich S, Sartor A. Cyproterone acetate and meningioma: a nationwide population-based study. J Neurooncol. Jan 2021;151(2):331-8.

16.   Bachir S, Shah S, Shapiro S, Koehler A, Mahammedi A, Samy RN, et al. Neurofibromatosis Type 2 (NF2) and the Implications for Vestibular Schwannoma and Meningioma Pathogenesis. Int J Mol Sci. 12 Jan 2021;22(2):690.

17.   Champeaux C, Wilson E, Brandner S, Shieff C, Thorne L. World Health Organization grade III meningiomas. A retrospective study for outcome and prognostic factors assessment. Br J Neurosurg. 3 Sep 2015;29(5):693-8.

18.   Peart R, Melnick K, Cibula J, Walbert T, Gerstner ER, Rahman M, et al. Clinical management of seizures in patients with meningiomas: Efficacy of surgical resection for seizure control and patient-tailored postoperative anti-epileptic drug management. NeuroOncol Adv. June 3, 2023;5(Suppl 1):i58-66.

19.   Alruwaili AA, De Jesus O. Meningioma. In: StatPearls [Internet]. Treasure Island (FL): StatPearls Publishing; 2024 [cited 2024 Feb 7]. Available from: http://www.ncbi.nlm.nih.gov/books/NBK560538/

20.   Huang RY, Bi WL, Griffith B, Kaufmann TJ, la Fougère C, Schmidt NO, et al. Imaging and diagnostic advances for intracranial meningiomas. Neuro-Oncol. Jan 14, 2019;21(Suppl 1):i44-61.

21.   behzadmehr R, behzadmehr R. Are the clinical manifestations of CT scan and location associated with World Health Organization histopathological grades of meningioma: A retrospective study. Ann Med Surg. Apr 30, 2021;66:102365.

22.   Kunimatsu A, Kunimatsu N, Kamiya K, Katsura M, Mori H, Ohtomo K. Variants of meningiomas: a review of imaging findings and clinical features. Jpn J Radiol. 1 Jul 2016;34(7):459-69.

23.   Kawahara Y, Nakada M, Hayashi Y, Kai Y, Hayashi Y, Uchiyama N, et al. Prediction of high-grade meningioma by preoperative MRI assessment. J Neurooncol. May 2012;108(1):147-52.

24.   Surov A, Gottschling S, Mawrin C, Prell J, Spielmann RP, Wienke A, et al. Diffusion- Weighted Imaging in Meningioma: Prediction of Tumor Grade and Association with Histopathological Parameters. Transl Oncol. Dec 2015;8(6):517-23.

25.   Zhang H, Rodiger LA, Shen T, Miao J, Oudkerk M. Perfusion MR imaging for differentiation of benign and malignant meningiomas. Neuroradiology. 2008;50(6):525-30.

26.   Watts J, Box G, Galvin A, Brotchie P, Trost N, Sutherland T. Magnetic resonance imaging of meningiomas: a pictorial review. Insights Imaging. feb 2014;5(1):113-22.

27.   Tamrazi B, Shiroishi MS, Liu CSJ. Advanced Imaging of Intracranial Meningiomas. Neurosurg Clin N Am. Apr 2016;27(2):137-43.

28.   Palma L, Celli P, Franco C, Cervoni L, Cantore G. Long-term prognosis for atypical and malignant meningiomas: a study of 71 surgical cases. J Neurosurg. May 1997;86(5):793-800.

29.   Sughrue ME, Sanai N, Shangari G, Parsa AT, Berger MS, McDermott MW. Outcome and survival following primary and repeat surgery for World Health Organization Grade III meningiomas: Clinical article. J Neurosurg. August 1, 2010;113(2):202-9.

30.   Chen WC, Perlow HK, Choudhury A, Nguyen MP, Mirchia K, Youngblood MW, et al. Radiotherapy for meningiomas. J Neurooncol. 2022;160(2):505-15.

31.   Bertero L, Dalla Dea G, Osella-Abbate S, Botta C, Castellano I, Morra I, et al. Prognostic Characterization of Higher-Grade Meningiomas: A Histopathological Score to Predict Progression and Outcome. J Neuropathol Exp Neurol. March 2019;78(3):248-56.

32.   Tjuatja F, Handoko null, Kodrat H, Yunus RE, Susanto E, Anindhita T, et al. Correlation of Ki-67 with Radiation Response and Grade in Meningiomas: A Systematic Review. Gulf J Oncolog. Sept 2022;1(40):58-66.

33.   Goldbrunner R, Stavrinou P, Jenkinson MD, Sahm F, Mawrin C, Weber DC, et al. EANO guideline on the diagnosis and management of meningiomas. Neuro-Oncol. Nov 2, 2021;23(11):1821-34.

34.   Dziuk TW, Woo S, Butler EB, Thornby J, Grossman R, Dennis WS, et al. Malignant meningioma: an indication for initial aggressive surgery and adjuvant radiotherapy. J Neurooncol. Apr 1998;37(2):177-88.

35.   institut national du cancer. Conduites à tenir devant des patients atteints d'un méningiome de grade II et III / Thésaurus [Internet]. 2020. Disponible sur: file:///C:/Users/Nesrine/Downloads/Conduites%20%C3%A0%20tenir%20M%C3%A9ningi omes%20-%20th%C3%A9saurus%20-%20sept%2020%20(6).pdf

36.   Chan AW, Bernstein KD, Adams JA, Parambi RJ, Loeffler JS. Dose Escalation with Proton Radiation Therapy for High-Grade Meningiomas. Technol Cancer Res Treat. Dec 1, 2012;11(6):607-14.

37.   Moazzam AA, Wagle N, Zada G. Recent developments in chemotherapy for meningiomas: a review. Neurosurg Focus. Dec 2013;35(6):E18.

38.   Sci-Hub | Emerging clinical imaging techniques for cerebral cavernous malformations: a systematic review | 10.3171/2010.5.FOCUS10120 [Internet]. [cited 18 Feb 2021]. Available from: https://scihub.wikicn.top/10.3171/2010.5.FOCUS10120

39.   Walcott BP, Nahed BV, Brastianos PK, Loeffler JS. Radiation Treatment for WHO Grade II and III Meningiomas. Front Oncol [Internet]. 2013 [cited 20 Feb 2024];3. Available from:

https://www.frontiersin.org/journals/oncology/articles/10.3389/fonc.2013.00227

40.   Zhao P, Li N, Cao J, Lin X, Liang C. Rhabdoid Meningioma Arising Concurrent in Pulmonary and Intracranial with a Rare Malignant Clinical Progression: Case Report and Literature Review. World Neurosurg. nov 2017;107:1046.e17-1046.e22.

41.   Surov A, Gottschling S, Bolz J, Kornhuber M, Alfieri A, Holzhausen HJ, et al. Distant metastases in meningioma: an underestimated problem. J Neurooncol. May 1, 2013;112(3):323-7.

42.   Ore CLD, Magill ST, Yen AJ, Shahin MN, Lee DS, Lucas CHG, et al. Meningioma metastases: incidence and proposed screening paradigm. J Neurosurg. Apr 5, 2019;132(5):1447-55.

43.   Villanueva-Meyer JE, Magill ST, Lee JC, Umetsu SE, Flavell RR. Detection of Metastatic Meningioma to the Liver Using 68Ga-DOTA-Octreotate PET/CT. Clin Nucl Med. Sept 2018;43(9):e338-40.

44.   Teague SD, Conces DJ. Metastatic meningioma to the lungs. J Thorac Imaging. Feb 2005;20(1):58-60.

45.   Corniola MV, Meling TR. Management of Recurrent Meningiomas: State of the Art and Perspectives. Cancers. August 18, 2022;14(16):3995.

46.   Maiuri F, Mariniello G, Guadagno E, Barbato M, Corvino S, Del Basso De Caro M. WHO grade, proliferation index, and progesterone receptor expression are different according to the location of meningioma. Acta Neurochir (Wien). Dec 1, 2019;161(12):2553-61.

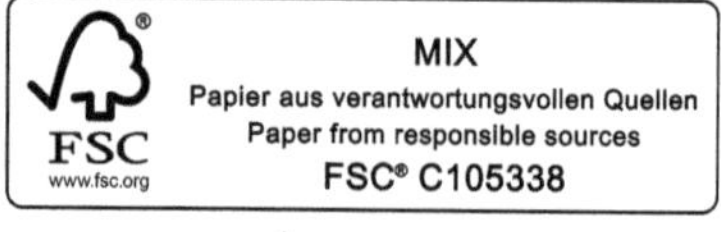

Printed by Books on Demand GmbH, Norderstedt / Germany